Homemade Hair Treatments: All Natural DIY Recipes that Promote Healthy and Beautiful Hair (Shampoos, Conditioners, and Hair Growth)

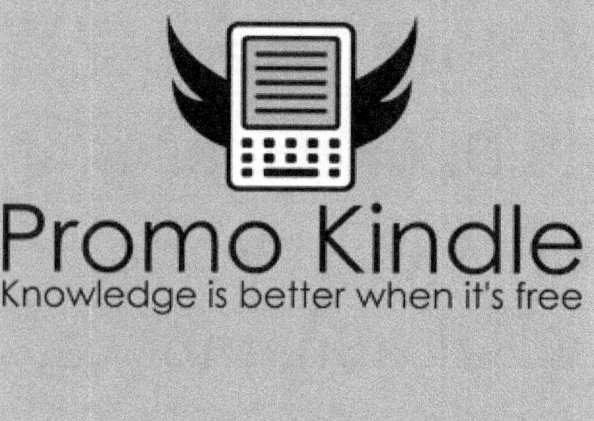

Disclaimer and Terms of Use: Effort has been made to ensure that the information in this book is accurate and complete, however, the author and the publisher do not warrant the accuracy of the information, text and graphics contained within the book due to the rapidly changing nature of science, research, known and unknown facts and internet. The Author and the publisher do not hold any responsibility for errors, omissions or contrary interpretation of the subject matter herein. This book is presented solely for motivational and informational purposes only.

Table of Contents

Shampoos

Moisturizing shampoo

Ingredient:

- 1 C Castile soap (liquid)
- ¼ C olive oil
- 1/8 C honey

Mix everything together and pour into air tight container or clean shampoo bottle

Vegan Shampoo

Ingredients:

- 1 C water
- 1 C liquid castile
- 2 T grapeseed
- 1/8 C aloe vera
- 5 drops essential oil, fragrance of your choice

Mix everything together and add to squeezable bottle

Conditioner

Ingredients:
- 2 C water
- ½ C apple cider vinegar

Mix ingredients together and add to squeezable bottle

Curly Hair Cleanser

Ingredients:
- 1 gallon brewed tea
- ½ C baking soda
- ¼ C castile soap
- 3 T xanthan gum
- 30 Drops essential oils

Directions: Let the tea cool, and then you can add the remaining ingredients and let sit and thicken (not too much) transfer to your preferred shampoo bottle

Coconut Milk Shampoo

Ingredients:
- ¼ C coconut milk
- 1/3 C organic baby shampoo
- 1 tsp vitamin E or almond oil
- 15 drops essential oils

Mix everything together well and store in shampoo bottles.

Clean Scalp Treatment recipe

Ingredients:
- 1 can coconut milk
- 1 ¾ C aloe vera gel

Directions: mix both ingredients in a large bowl and whisk until they are well mixed well. Pour the mix into ice cube trays and let freeze. When your ready to use one, let it thaw before use, and use it like normal shampoo.

Lice Remedies Recipes

Coconut Oil

Ingredients:
- apple cider vinegar
- Coconut oil

Directions: start with rinsing your hair in apple cider vinegar, and let it dry. Now saturate head and scald hair, everything with coconut oil and cover with a cap or plastic bag. You will need to leave this on for a full 8 hours or overnight is even better. In the morning, comb thru your hair carefully, then wash with regular shampoo.

Sesame Seed Oil recipe

Ingredients:
- ¼ C sesame seed oil
- 1/8 tsp tee tree oil
- ½ tsp euayptus & rosemary oil
- 10 drops lavender oil

Directions: Mix above ingredients together in small to medium size bowl, and rinse hair with apple cider vinegar and let dry. Add the oil blend to hair and cover. Let sit overnight than shampoo and rinse as normal.

Garlic treatment

Ingredients:
- 8-10 garloc clove or minced garlic
- 3 T lime juice
- Hot water

Directions: If you are using whole cloves, you need to grind them up. It needs to be a paste like consistency with the lime juice add rub into the scalp and leave on for about 30-45 minutes. Rinse

Tea tree treatment

Ingredients:
- 1 T tea tree oil
- 1 oz. regular shampoo
- 3 T coconut

Directions: Mix everything together and apply throughout your hair and scalp. Cover your head and leave on for about an hour to an hour and a half. Rinse thoroughly with HOT water and you want to comb thru to remove the nasty dead lice.

Hair growth shampoo recipes

Honey Shampoo

Ingredients:
- Raw honey
- Essential oils
- Water

Directions: This is a single serve recipe, because you don't want them to go bad. Add everything together and pour into container or bowl. You want to use this after you make it. You can store it for a few days in a small shampoo bottle.

Herbal Shampoo Recipe

Ingredients:
- 2 oz. mild castile soap
- 4 ½ oz water
- ¼ tsp carrier oil
- 30 drops essential oil

Directions: you can add a herbal diffusion to your ater for aroma. This is optional. You want use a heat proof jar, let simmer with the herbs and cap the car, letting it marinade. Add the castile soap oil and essential oils to your water and stir gently. You don't want a whole lot of bubbles if possible. Pour into old recycled shampoo bottle or any $1 bottle from your local Dollar store works as well.

Dandruff Shampoo recipe

Ingredients:
- 2 aspirin crushed
- Normal shampoo 1-2 T

Directions: Crush the tablets until they are like powder and add them to the 2-3 T of normal shampoo. Use this for a few days.

Dry Shampoo

Ingredients:
- 2 T arrowroot powder
- 2 T cocoa powder
- Combine ingredients and you can store them in a mason jar or other jar that has a lid, you want to keep this dry.

All natural Stress relieving shampoo

Ingredients:
- 10 oz. mineral water
- 2 chamomile tea bags
- 24 oz. almond oil
- 2 oz. beeswax
- 2 oz. creamed coconut
- 4 oz. caustic soda
- 4 T essential oil
- 2 tsp essential oil
- 1 tsp essential oil
- 1 tsp rosemary essential oil

Directions: Add chamomile teabags in saucepan and boil water, strain and let cool. Melt coconut and wax and oils. Combine everything together. You want everything to simmer together for a while, don't let things sit on the bottom for too long. Pour into ice cube trays and let sit. Like wax you want these to harden.

Conditioners

Basic Conditioner

Ingredients:
- 1 tsp carrier oil coconut oil
- 1 tsp vegetable sugar
- 1 T emulsifying wax
- ½ tsp vitamin E
- ½ C water
- 5 tsp. grapefruit extract
- Essential oils

Directions: stir oil, wax, and sugar wax in double boiler over low heat until wax melts. Remove from direct heat and add your Vitamin E. Separate bowls start slowly warming the water, You just want is.. Barely warm, lukewarm would be fine. Pour the water into the oil mixture. And wick you want this smooth. You don't want these separating too fast, that is why you need to WHISK instead of just stirring. Stir in the essential oils and grapefruit. You can pour this into a small glass bottle or plastic squeeze bottle. You want this to cool before you pour into the bottle of course. Shake before using.

Ingredients:
- 2 C water
- Herbs (chamomile, green tea, peppermint or other preferred herb)

Directions: Bring water and herbs to a boil, remove for heat and let sit for about an hour. Strain the herbs from the water and add 2 T apple cider vinegar.

Ingredients:
- 1 VERY RIPE banana
- 2 T extra virgin olive oil
- ¼ C T plain greek yogurt
- 1 T raw honey
- Hair cap

Directions: Move the olive oil and banana to the blender and blenduntil very smooth. Add remaining ingredients and mix well, you don't want a whole lot of lumps. Obviously. You can use a strainer to remove extra lumps. You want to make this before using, this isn't the kind of conditioner you want to store for too long.

Green Conditioner

Ingredients:
- 1 mashed avocado
- 2 T organic honey
- 1 T extra virgin olive oil

Directions: Probably best to add the avocado to the blender JUST ot be sure its "mashed" very well and smooth. Then add your remaining ingredients and add those to the blender as well, and blend again, until very smooth. Add to wet hair, cover with a cap and let it sit for about an hour then rinse.

Ingredients:
- 1 C plain greek yogurt
- 1 T castor oil
- 1 T coconut oil
- 1 whipped egg

Directions: Use a medium size bowl, whip your yogurt and add rest of the ingredients, that simple. Apply to your wet/damp hair and leave on for about an hour and rinse.

Cure for Dandruff Conditioner

Ingredients:
- 1 C plain Greek yogurt
- ¼ C sesame oil
- 2 T aloe Vera gel
- 1 T olive oil
- 3 drops tea tree oil

Directions: Whip everything together until everything is smooth and apply to damp hair, let it sit for about an hour or longer than rinse

Ingredients
- 1 C regular mayo
- 1/3 C yogurt
- 1/3 C coconut oil
- 2 T honey

Directions: mix everything together and make sure its all well blended and apply to wet hair, let sit for about an hour or longer then rinse thoroughly.

Color Treated Drinks

Ingredients:
- 1-3 T shampoo
- 1-3 T conditioner
- 4 Oz spritz bottle with beer

Directions: wash and condition your hair as normal then spritz the beer on your hair before blow drying. This treats color treated hair.

Dark Hair treatment

Ingredients:
- 1 oz. dried root
- Comfrey root
- Sage leaf
- 15 oz. Olive oil
- 3 oz. herbal infused olive oil

Directions: cool and cover the above ingredients, then you will add this to your hair as a deep conditioning treatment.

Banana avocados

Ingredients:
- Avocado and divided
- 1-2 ripe bananas

Directions: combine both and blend until smooth, add to hair and leave on for 15 minutes then rinse.